Constipation

Or everything you need to know about bowel peristalsis

Constantin Panow

"Every soldier has in his bag the marshal's rod."

General Aleksandr Vasilyevich Suvorov

Russian Field Marshall, 1729-1800

A frequent issue in general medicine, coprostasis isn't an innocuous subject.

Diverticulitis, and acute appendicitis are most feared complications.

Apart from its infectious counterpart, common problem is bloating, abdominal fullness, and general discomfort.

Psychology

Being related to poor mood, a constipated person is considered uninteresting and dull.

Dryness

Especially in hot summer months, when temperature is high and people don't drink enough, this is a frequent consultation reason.

Winter season is less concerned, unless there is overheating of one's flat.

Despite simple and easy treatment and prevention available, especially in industrialized countries, medical attention remains high.

Intestinal movement

In recent years professional community acknowledged a huge advance in this area, recognizing that fiber-carbohydrates, which is vegetables make bowel peristalsis not faster, but slower.

In American gastroenterology it is known since two centuries, that starch-carbohydrates ferment faster than fiber-carbohydrates.

Modernity

Thus, now we are at last able to have a more complete image of this topic.

Here I need to present a short survey of nutriments and their digestion.

Nowadays literature separates carbohydrates (CH) in fiber-CH, which is vegetables and green salad, as previously mentioned and starches-CH, which is bread, pasta, rice, and other cereals, and potatoes.

Fruit is to be considered separately, as it contains and liberates mainly fructose.

Apart from that, we should examine proteins, which is cheese, meat, poultry, and fish.

We should deal singly with oils and fats.

Bowel movements, which is peristalsis and its speed is determined by fine neuro-humoral interactions represented by nerves and hormones.

If we start proximally, that is with esophagus, there isn't a lot to be said about this organ in this respect.

In contradistinction to stomach, the emptying of which is highly variable on content.

As soon as alimentary encompassing reaches proximal small bowel by action of vagus nerve, there is release of many small intestinal peptides, cholecystokinin and secretin for instance, to name only a few, which slow down stomach emptying.

Small bowel

This action is essential to make digestion possible by gastric, pancreatic and liver juices.

As you can suppose already from previous discussion, more energetic food is admitted to duodenum in a more sluggish way, than low-energy one.

So, starches-CH, which are digested almost immediately into L-glucose, are most tremendous promoter of this action, of slowing down of stomach peristalsis, and especially if ingested at the same time as proteins. (Even more so if oils are added.)

Fruit, releasing fructose, is next on the list, and last are, of course fiber-CH, fats staying somewhere in between.

As already discussed, starches-CH are digested fast to L-glucose, but not only that, they lose bulk substantially in their travel to colon.

They are also main promoter of flatus.

In contradistinction fiber-CHs ferment little, as they need appropriate germs for that action, remain with a lot of bulk when they reach large bowel, and are better hydrated.

They are digested into D-glucose, and release this nutriment continuously through bowel migration.

Distal small bowel

Not unlikely to this, fruit releases fructose only slowly, and attains ileum with high energetic content, which boosts serotonin release from distal intestine, (vermiform appendix, colon and ileum), and activates progress in large bowel most efficiently. (As well as equilibrating mood- CNS action).

Fruit

From previous expose it results, that most efficient anti-coprostasis operation is unfolded by fruit.

Fiber-CH come next, while starches-CH have a constipating force.

Intestinal juices are least important of all water body volume for immediate homeostasis and thus are depleted fastest on drink restriction: - Coprostasis is consequence!

Movement

Neuro-vegetative system plays an important role in peristalsis, with its parasympathetic part, stimulating, and sympathetic counterpart, with an inhibiting movement.

Their response is reliant on general physical activity.

Thus, I propose at least one hour of walking every day to my patients.

Hydration

Drinking two liters of liquid every day, or till diuresis is abundant, is also relevant for our purpose.

MLM

As to general dietetic advice, concerning starches-CH, I propose a French proverb: -"Mange la moitié!" MLM or "Eat half!"

Replacing these with fiber-CH.

Fruit in good quantity is essential, but if you are reluctant to eat too much sweet, as I am, you can limit yourself to one pear every day, to my opinion this one being the best ingredient for our intent.

Other ones are figs and plums, but the season for these two is short.

Hence you can prepare yourself a mush of dried fruit, most important being last mentioned two.

You cut them into small pieces, cover them with hot water in a pot and let them simmer gently for half an hour. You can add cinnamon, lemon in pieces and vanilla to make this compote more palatable. Don't add sugar! -This would be excessive.

Intestinal flora

Last, but not least, I would like to entertain you with some measures to balance of germs in your intestine.

They are present everywhere in bowel, dominant in large one, while stomach content being because of its acid almost sterile.

To be in good shape it is essential to take care of this aspect.

Coming from Bulgaria, I advise my patients to eat some yoghurt every single day.

A bit of molded cheese, like gorgonzola, would have a similar action.

Another European specialty is Sauerkraut, which

should be consumed raw. (If possible bio)

To render it appetizing, add some water, mix it well, till it's not too sour!

Then separate the juice and drink it apart.

Beware! It is laxative.

With the rest of the Sauerkraut you can prepare salad to be enjoyed with paprika and vegetable oil.

One or two raw tomatoes (possibly bio) per day add lections to colon, which level bacteria there.

Green bananas and chicory (the drink) have a similar action.

Sugars are to be avoided, as they promote infection, tumor, and diabetes, obesity and so forth.

Bad ones are to be avoided, and easiest way is through nutritional measures.

Quercetin present in spring onions, tomatoes, especially bio, and green salad has an important action in this respect.

Resveratrol, contained in red, or dark grapes and red wine, gives a similar response.

But, most important of all is raw garlic. One to two cloves in the evening should be enough.

If you are suffering from germ infestation, for instance Candida albicans, you should follow this advice at all time.

Otherwise, taking it on week-ends should be

enough.

Curcuma is another agent employed against mushrooms.

It should be consumed with black pepper or ginger to render it absorbable through bowel wall.

This recipe is efficient also against nail mycosis and Herpes.

Exceptions

Most fruit has a laxative action, big exceptions being ripe bananas and blueberries, which are constipating.

I hope you enjoyed this short text.

I am convinced that observing above measures from time to time would have a positive effect on your general well-being and health.

Internet

You can reach me at my site:

www.thenopillshealthprospect.com

If you have questions or comments, don't hesitate, write in my blog!